DEDICATION

This book is dedicated to Lily. You are the light of my life. You are the reason I wake up every morning. Please stay as beautiful and wonderful forever.

TABLE OF CONTENTS

Don't Forget Your Mental Health

How to Strengthen Your Conscious and Subconscious Minds

By: Kevin Green

9781635019919

PUBLISHERS NOTES

Disclaimer – Speedy Publishing LLC

This publication is intended to provide helpful and informative material. It is not intended to diagnose, treat, cure, or prevent any health problem or condition, nor is intended to replace the advice of a physician. No action should be taken solely on the contents of this book. Always consult your physician or qualified health-care professional on any matters regarding your health and before adopting any suggestions in this book or drawing inferences from it.

The author and publisher specifically disclaim all responsibility for any liability, loss or risk, personal or otherwise, which is incurred as a consequence, directly or indirectly, from the use or application of any contents of this book.

Any and all product names referenced within this book are the trademarks of their respective owners. None of these owners have sponsored, authorized, endorsed, or approved this book.

Always read all information provided by the manufacturers' product labels before using their products. The author and publisher are not responsible for claims made by manufacturers.

This book was originally printed before 2014. This is an adapted reprint by Speedy Publishing LLC with newly updated content designed to help readers with much more accurate and timely information and data.

Speedy Publishing LLC

40 E Main Street, Newark, Delaware, 19711

Contact Us: 1-888-248-4521

Website: http://www.speedypublishing.co

REPRINTED Paperback Edition: 9781635019919:

Manufactured in the United States of America

Chapter 1- Mental Health and Professional Help

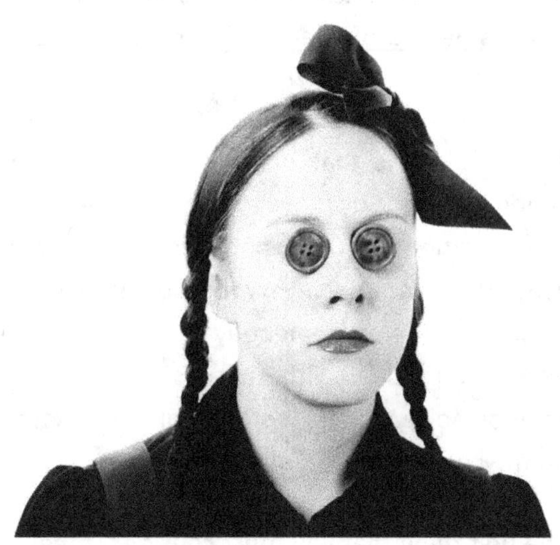

Many people are confused by mental illness and many will claim that they simply do not exist, that the condition is caused by the person experiencing it. However, everyday there are counselors who are diagnosing people as having mental illness conditions and because of this it makes it difficult to determine whether or not a diagnosis is correct. Also, because of this, there are many controversies surrounding these conditions.

Mental health is essential for everyday life. Most people are able to go through life without any glitches in their mental process, but others seem to have constant interruptions. It is these interruptions that show us that there is something going wrong in the brain of these individuals and that there is an existing problem. We need to look at different diagnoses and symptoms to understand the interruptions that occur in the brain.

For example, we should take bipolar depression as an example. This is one of the most common disorders diagnosed in today's society. In fact, you probably know somebody with bipolar depression you just don't know that they have it. Bipolar is very common, but many people don't fully understand the condition. Bipolar is a chemical imbalance in the brain. This means that the brain is denied of vital nutrients that it needs to maintain a stable mindset.

The problem is that many people who are diagnosed with the condition do not have their full life experiences taken into consideration. We all experience stress, trauma and drama in our lives. However, not everybody deals with these stressors in the same manner as somebody else would and nobody should be expected to deal with these stressors in the same manner as someone else would. There is a process that takes place that brings on the condition of bipolar depression.

The first thing that you must consider is that we all have "triggers." These triggers are the stressful events that happen in life. Now, everybody deals with these differently. Some people will respond negatively and others ignore. Those individuals who ignore these issues are often not hearing the messages in between. This is what separates the mentally ill mind from the "normal" mind.

The mentally ill mind tends to absorb everything in life that is said. They hear it all and they let all of that process in their brains until it begins to cause confusion. The "normal" mind tends to only listen to what it wants to listen to and therefore they do not have these conflicting thoughts to cause the mental confusion. To better understand this process, it helps to also understand cognitive mental health disorders and how these are related to the confusion that occurs in the mind.

Kevin Green
Cognitive Mental Health Disorders

Cognitive health disorders include:

•Dementia

•Delirium

•Alcohol-induced disorders

There are also several others that are related and all of these are constantly being studied so that we may gain a better understanding of them. Most of these disorders have several common denominators such as loss of memory. Others are linked brain and biological disease, such as alcoholism and drug addiction.

Often people who suffer from cognitive disorders have issues with reasoning and often their speech. They tend to lack good judgment and their comprehension is different from the "normal" mind.

These individuals also tend to suffer from other conditions such as:

•Depression

•Irritation

•Paranoia

There are several other related symptoms that are easily misdiagnosed with other conditions, such as bipolar, as bipolar condition encompasses several of these symptoms as well.

Delirium is one that is often confused because it includes:

•Signals confusion

•Speech problems

•Loss of memory

•Fear

•Depression

Many of these same symptoms are apparent in other mental illnesses, but delirium also has several physical effects on the body as well such as:

•Increased heart rate

•Nausea

•Disturbance in sleep

All of these physical symptoms as well as the mental confusion cause the person to not be able to find comfort in their life. Many studies have shown that medications can increase their symptoms as well to the point that the physical symptoms express themselves in strokes and heart attacks.

Dementia is a type of Alzheimer's disease. This causes the person to have issues with memory retention as well as learning and language. There are several physical conditions that can cause the onset of dementia such as AIDS, strokes, heart failures and other chronic conditions.

People that suffer from dementia also tend to suffer in personal hygiene and poor judgment as well. They tend to avoid others, alter their personality and have social anxiety in general. Many are manic depressive and should completely avoid alcohol.

Mentally ill patients tend to resort to drugs and alcohol and this only increases the symptoms of their condition and makes it worse, although it provides them temporary relief from their pain and suffering. However, alcohol and drugs are not a solution to anything in life and should be completely avoided by these individuals, as they are not likely to be able to keep their drinking at a social level.

There are alcohol induced disorders that have been classified as cognitive disorders because of the similar symptoms. In most of these cases the condition is a direct result of the condition, although this is not true of all individuals. Many individuals who are mentally ill have never touched drugs and alcohol, although many therapists will try to use alcohol and drugs as a reason for their condition. Those disorders that are alcohol induced are referred to as "Korsakoff's Syndrome" and it main affects the memory directly.

Symptoms of this condition include:

•Memory loss

•Denial

•Indifferences

•Violent behaviors

Most of these conditions can be directly linked to nutritional deficiencies because the alcoholic and drug user tend to not live very healthy and eat poorly. Alcoholism is difficult to treat, but it is possible. However, it does require a lot of diligence by the patient and they must accept that they have a problem in order for recovery to occur.

There are medications and treatments that can be used to assist the person and many will need therapy with high dosages of B-complex vitamins. If the patient is still in the early stages of alcoholism it will be easier to treat them as long as they are willing. Alcoholism is a very serious condition and it even affects children. Therapists are constantly looking for new ways to treat mental illness. There are millions of individuals around the world who suffer from mental illnesses and many rarely receive the care that they should.

Causes of Mental Health Problems

There are several different types of mental illnesses and all have a root that prompts them to manifest somewhere in a person's life. There are various conditions that people may suffer from including:

•Adjustment disorders

•Bipolar

•Sexual disorders

•Dementia

•Delirium

•Manic Depression

Adjustment disorders are common when a person has a hard time adapting to stress in their life. Bipolar is another common disorder that is often diagnosed in individuals, but this condition can easily be misconstrued and can be misdiagnosed.

Bipolar or manic depression affects individuals and often includes symptoms such as:

•Hyperactivity

•Excessive worrying

•Mood swings

These individuals seem to go from extreme highs to extreme lows in just a matter of minutes. They can literally drive a person crazy if they are not treated immediately. These individuals often threaten suicide, although many are just looking for attention and never actually attempt suicide. This condition is directly linked to a chemical imbalance in the brain and the condition is more neurological than physiological. This condition also has been linked to genetics and is likely to be passed on in a family. Many patients that have been diagnosed have a family history of similar behavior and mood swings.

Many of these chemical disorders are often linked back to childhood development and trauma that the person sustained and never received treatment for. If the trauma is allowed to fester and the person never has to accept and deal with it, bipolar symptoms will occur. Sexual disorders also occur in a similar way. These disorders are separate from bipolar and other adjustment disorders.

Sexual deviation is often linked to abuse, although not always, pornography, and other types of negative sexual behaviors. Recent studies have proven, however, that serial killers and sociopath behaviors are hereditary. Some studies have linked these conditions to child abuse and this may be the case in some instances, but not necessary all instances. Sexual disorders are psychological and there have been links of brain impairments that cause interruptions in the brain's processes which cause this behavior to manifest itself.

Dementia and delirium are mind disorders that tend to manifest themselves in older individuals. These cause memory loss and confusion. These can be tricky to diagnose if the patient is young as the condition could be caused by other illnesses in young individuals.

When Should You Ask For Professional Help

If you or a family member or friend is in therapy there are questions you should ask to avoid problems. The expertise levels of therapists do vary and not all are qualified to diagnose mental illness. If you suspect that you have a disorder you should do your best to be very accurate on your symptoms, research them and document them.

If you go to a therapist you will be ahead of the game and by knowing and researching your symptoms you may be able to prevent an incorrect diagnosis. When you visit a therapist they will talk to you and listen to you. They will search for many signs and disturbances in your thinking patterns.

Therapists will search for symptoms such as:

•Vague thoughts

•Fleeting ideas

•Peripheral thought patterns

•Blocking thoughts

•Disassociation

•Break in reality

•Paranoia

If the patient displays a disturbance in their thinking patterns, the therapist may consider psychosis. Counselors will consider schizophrenia or psychosis if the patient shows a break in reality. Paranoid and paranoia may be misconstrued if the therapist doesn't have a good understanding between the two conditions.

Schizophrenics are often paranoid and may suffer from posttraumatic stress in the early stages. If a patient provides answers to questions that are unrelated, the therapist may consider a potential mental illness. Another area of concern is if the patient speaks in fragments of thoughts and don't deliver complete sentences or ideas. This is known as a fleeting thought process. If a patient is illustrating thoughts that are off the subject, the therapist may also show concern.

Other areas that are considered include language. Some patients may simply have a lack of education, but they should be able to speak in a comprehensible manner. It is important that the patient is not misdiagnosed simply because they have poor communication skills. Because every person is different and may have a different level of education it is important that that the therapist pay attention to symptoms that are linked to mental health. Be certain to ask the therapist questions any time there is a diagnosis and what the diagnosis is based on.

For example, if the patient is telling the therapist about a dream and all of a sudden can't remember what they are talking about, this can be an evident that the patient has suffered trauma. The symptoms are in front of the therapist, but it is wise to continue therapy to verify the diagnosis.

Many therapists are not trained sufficiently in certain conditions, such as Multiple Personality Disorder. These conditions require you to carefully examine the person because they may only be suffering from dementia. However, if they are suffering from Multiple Personality Disorder it is often because they are trying to block traumatic memories to avoid pain. It is always wise to ask questions when you are visiting a therapist and this can also help them to avoid any mistakes.

A healthy mind is important and mental health should not be taken lightly. Therapists are constantly studying the mind and often use the guinea pig method until they figure out what the issue is. Mental health symptoms are serious and should not be taken lightly.

matters even more, the judicial system seems to have its own version of what these conditions are as well.

Some of the most common symptoms of alcoholism and drug abuse include:

•Excessive drinking/drugging

•Problems with the law

•Withdrawal symptoms

•Shaking of hands

If a person drinks daily and relies on alcohol, then you are most likely dealing with an alcoholic. Although, everyone seems to have their own definition of what an alcohol is, but the bottom line is that withdrawal symptoms manifest themselves and the person needs alcohol to relieve them then they are an alcoholic, no matter what time of the day they have their first drink. Each person is different physically in how they deal with alcohol as well. If you started drinking when you were young and you have been able to drink without alcohol causing you any issues then you are probably not an alcoholic.

The fact is that alcoholism and drug addiction are very complex conditions. Alcohol and drugs become a problem when the person is unable to control their use and increases their intake and then combines the two. If someone will steal or lie to obtain alcohol then they are likely addicted. Many people with other mental illnesses will also resort to alcohol and drugs to find relief from their symptoms.

Chapter 2- How Substance Abuse Affects the Mental Health

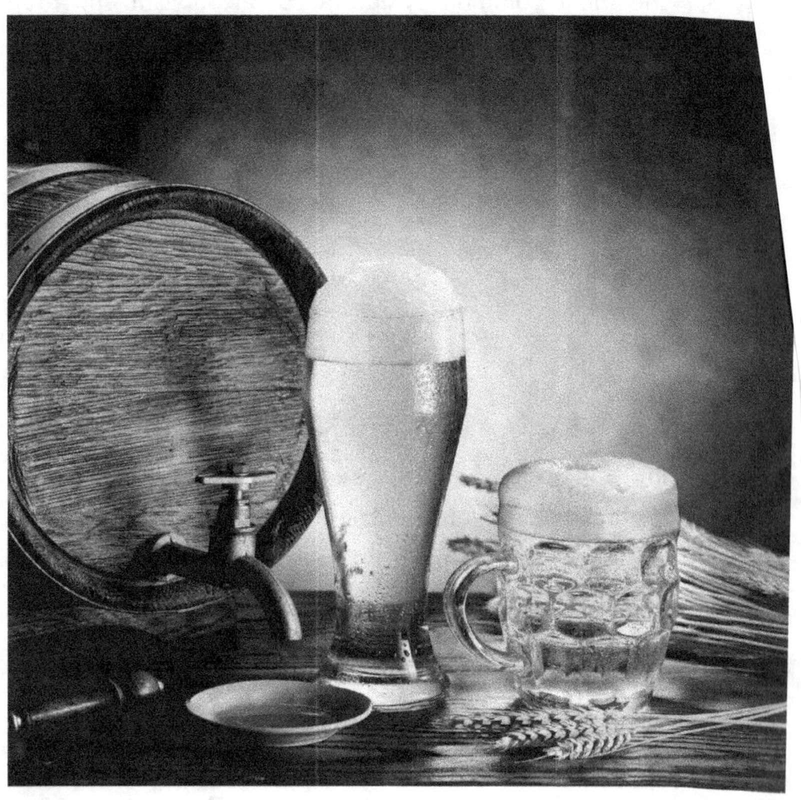

Alcohol and Drug Abuse

There are several mental illnesses and scientists are constantly searching to understand the various mental illnesses that exist. Here we will discover just a few of the most common illnesses in detail.

Alcohol abuse and drug abuse are two conditions that are both very serious. However, it seems that alcoholism often gets more attention than drug abuse, when drug abuse should often be looked at more closely. The DSM manual suggests that there are actually differences in the definition of both conditions. To confuse

Alcoholism and drug addiction are conditions that can be treated and overcome but it does require a lot of motivation to quit on the person's behalf. Many people must first hit rock bottom before they are willing to admit that they have a problem and many people are never able to admit they have a problem and there is little hope for these individuals.

You can't make a person quit drinking or doing drugs, but you can support them once they have taken it upon themselves to quit.

Antisocial and Psychopathic Disorders

To diagnose antisocial and psychopathic disorders, mental health experts first use the Conduct Control Behaviors or Disorders rules to diagnose a patient over the age of 18 with Antisocial Personality Disorder. This particular disorder often has several underlying disorders that can mimic other symptoms to cause a false diagnosis.

These symptoms may include, but are not limited to:

• Fire starting and pyromania

• Truancy

• Theft

• Harming of people

• Harming and killing small animals

• Hostility towards authority

• Violent outbursts

•Dangerous sexual acts

•Willful or malicious destruction of property

•Compulsive-implosive explosions

•Crime

There are many more symptoms related to this condition, but quite frankly many are very frightening. Psychopathic symptoms are very similar to those above and include:

•Fire starting

•Bed wetting

•Harming or killing people

•Harming or killing small animals

•Explosive outbursts

•Conduct control disorders

•Inability to regard others

•Destruction

•Truancy

•Neglectful attitude

•Sexual deviant behavior

•Hostility towards authority

Kevin Green
•Inability to show remorse

•Inability to express emotions

•Impulsive-compulsive behaviors

•Criminal minded

Individuals who suffer from antisocial and psychopathic conditions are unable to show emotion at all and they never show remorse for their actions. If they do show remorse, it is superficial and they really don't have any feelings of remorse at all.

These two areas of mental illness include the following illnesses:

•Antisocial personalities

•Sociopath personalities

•Histrionic personalities

•Psychopathic personalities

It is easy to see how these conditions can have a similar diagnosis, as they are related and linked quite closely in diagnosis. The differences are slight and in reality the two are very similar. These two conditions are often diagnosed and linked to each other in a condition called Psychopathic disorder with Antisocial Personality Disorder, Psychopathic traits and tendencies.

Because of the closeness in diagnosis, many mental health experts have conflicting opinions on Antisocial Personality Disorder, because it is essentially psychopathic. Psychopathic Personalities are up on reality, but their morals and social beliefs tend to determine their symptoms. These people often engage in sexual exploits and are more often affected by pornographic materials and pornographic materials are often the leading cause behind a psychopath's mind.

These conditions also have hereditary link and their behaviors are genetic. Also, although alcohol and drug use are common among these individuals, not all are alcoholics or drug addicts. Several individuals have been diagnosed with this condition and have never touched either substance. Many resort to these substances though to relieve the pain of their symptoms. These individuals do not always commit murder either. Many of those who do commit murder are those who have not been treated.

It may take years to work through the symptoms of these conditions, but in the long run you can work with them and treat them. This is important to stop these individuals from becoming serial killers. It is often the individuals who are never treated that resort to killing.

CHAPTER 3- MENTAL DISORDERS OF GENETIC ORIGINS

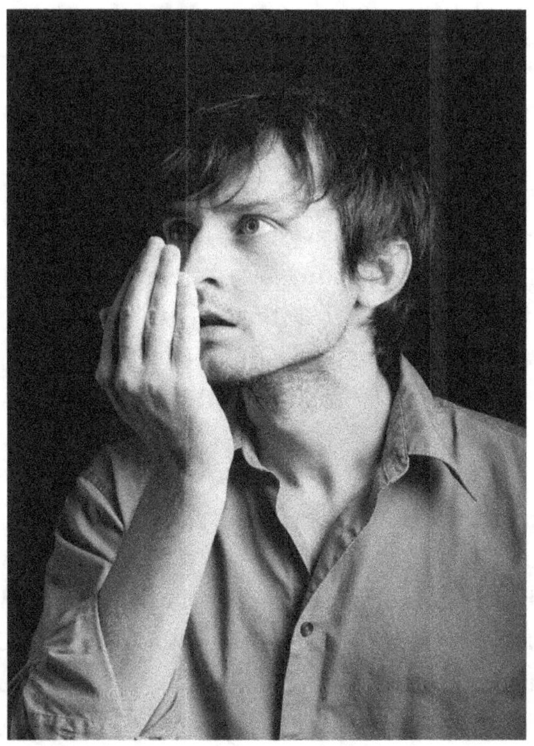

Avoidant Personality Disorder

Avoidant Personality Disorder is a personality type that will avoid the public due to a fear of rejection, disappointment, humiliation, and that people will view them as a failure. They are often reluctant to speak in public, ask for help or ask questions. These individuals also tend to work below their abilities, as being promoted is frightening to them.

Many of these individuals will also suffer from:

•Inferiority complexes

•Severe episodes of loneliness

•Depression

•Anxiety attacks

Schizoid personality types are similar to this condition; however, they will avoid public but still need to socialize. Avoidant Personality Disorder types do not have a desire to socialize at all. Avoidant personality types are easy to treat without medication because their symptoms are all rooted in fear. Therapeutic treatment can work through their fears by starting with the deepest fear the person displays. Through talk therapy, role play and other strategies, therapists can do wonders for avoidant personality disorders.

It is important to listen to these types, as the problem lies in their thoughts and concerns. When a person is telling someone that they have a problem with socialization, we know that underneath those words lies fear that is often caused by an incident or accident from their childhood. These individuals may have endured some underdevelopment or lack of education and knowledge as well because they stay under the radar in an attempt to not outperform others. If this person is taught or relearns the rules of society they can often socialize without problems. If a therapist can work through the problems without covering them up with medication then the person can come out of their shell.

Dependent Personality Disorder

Dependent Personality Disorders are common according to many mental health experts. These individuals suffer from symptoms such as:

- Incompetence to make their own decisions

- Rely on others to make decisions for them

- Avoid responsibility

- Rely on others to handle their lives and tasks

- Avoid tasks unless someone else guides them through the process.

- Tolerate abuse and neglect, including the cheating of a spouse

- Often depressed

- Often abuse alcohol and drugs to relieve anxiety

- Passive

- Will not defend themselves

- Afraid of rejection

- Afraid of punishment

It is important that these symptoms are carefully scrutinized and they should not be confused with women who are submissive, as the traditional woman will not tolerate anyone going against their beliefs and will defend their person without thinking twice.

Dependent personality types are found in individuals who have Histrionic and Borderline personality types. The difference is that Histrionic and Borderline personality types may be manipulative, controlling, and abusive and act out dangerously. These individuals can be manipulative and may even murder. The dependent personality type is not aggressive and can hold a relationship, while Histrionic and Borderline personality types cannot hold a relationship. Dependent personality types need ongoing therapy because they have underlying fear from undo punishment, neglect or abuse. The person most likely lived in an unruly home and received harsh punishment.

Most dependent types will rely on their parents to make their decisions for them and the parent often finds a reason to dismiss the decisions the person does make. For example, if the person was engaged in a relationship that broke up, the parent will tell them something like, "I told you so, that girl/boy was too good for you." They are constantly put down as not being able to make good decisions for themselves, so they rely on others to do it for them. These individuals will become so dependent that they begin to ask for permission for anything they do, even simple tasks like going to bed or going to the store. These people become co-dependent because their parents won't allow them to move forward in life. Therefore, the patient must separate him or herself so that they begin to develop their own independence.

Therapists must also use techniques that will work to help the patient separate from those that they are dependent upon and move towards relying on themselves. Most therapists will rely on talk therapy because the patient holds the answers, they just don't realize it because they are used to being told that they are wrong. In most instances we know that the patient was neglected or harshly punished often and often scolded. It is also useful to work through their mental problems.

You can talk through their problems and sort out the information to gather the background of the person's behavior. While working with these individuals the therapist should never raise their voice r attempt to control them. They must be allowed to speak freely and open up. Do not allow the person to blame his or herself as this only contributes to their dependency.

Schizophrenia

Schizophrenia is a condition that has plagued the mental health world for decades. Mental health experts have been finding more cases of these individuals than they have in the past. This condition is nothing that should be ignored and ignoring the diagnosis only adds to the problem. Schizophrenia has several levels of symptoms and these patients must be treated immediately.

Any person complaining of any of the following must receive treatment immediately:

•Paranoia

•Hallucinations

•Hearing voices

These individuals suffer immensely and those around them also suffer because of the person's actions and lack of reality. They often feel that someone is trying to get them or coming to get them. They may also tell you that the CIA or KGB is out to get them as well. Hallucinations affect the sensory in the sense that it conveys messages to sense organs and then creates a suspicious force.

This causes the person to be suspicious of everything around them including objects, places, things and people. Once they suspicion sets in they can become extremely dangerous and may act out violently. The twin area of the brain is affected in this condition and causes the individual to break off from reality.

Medication is often required to prevent schizophrenic episodes and hallucinations. Researchers have been astounded by this condition for years and are always seeking answers to questions regarding the condition. The hallucinations that these individuals suffer from are similar to psychotic breaks and the patient loses contact with reality. The voices that they hear often tell them that there is danger near, which is often not true.

An example of a serious schizophrenic was the Oklahoma City Bomber. Signs that a person may be schizophrenic include:

•Laughing for no apparent reason

•Shouting at the air

•Constant muttering during periodicals

•Covering ears

Most individuals who suffer from this condition are recognized by the age of 13 and these individuals are often not treated until later in life when they should be treated much earlier. This is often because certain symptoms are often found in other disorders and professionals wait to see if the person is a true schizophrenic or if they are suffering from another condition. The downside is that if the person is not treated early enough they often break into paranoia and this is when diagnosis is quite dangerous.

The reason is because they begin to hear voices in their head and they may claim the voices are from God, the Devil or aliens. Their visual perspective is often similar to the voices they hear in their head. They may tell you that they see people from the CIA or KGB or that someone delivered packages to their door, etc. These individuals are not typically suicidal, but would rather kill than die.

Kevin Green
There have been a few cases of schizophrenics showing suicidal behaviors however.

CHAPTER 4- DISORDERS COMMONLY SEEN IN CHILDREN

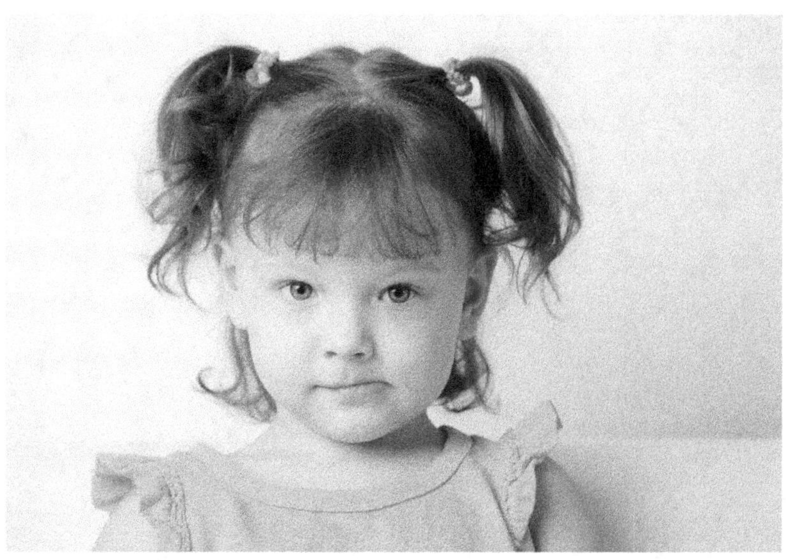

Auditory Processing Hyperactive Disorder (ADHD)

Auditory Processing Hyperactive Disorder is also known as Attention-Deficit Hyperactivity Disorder or better yet, ADHD. ADHD is a product of the misprocessing of the auditory stimuli and a hearing deficiency. Auditory Processing Hyperactive Disorder is coupled with Attention Deficit and Hypertension Disorder. Auditory Processing Hyperactive Disorder is most common in children and teenagers and not so much in adults.

However, adults have recently been diagnosed quite frequently as of late. Warning signs of this condition include:

•Incapacity to use common sense

•Verbalizes without caring about others

•Constantly feeling a great sense of boredom

•Lack of focus

•Act before thinking

•Disregard the consequences of their actions and behaviors

The cranial nerve that connects the inner ear with the brain transfers impulses that control balance and hearing. When the auditory process is interrupted, the person feel aggravated and becomes hyperactive. This leads to Attention Deficit Hyperactivity. These individuals seem to have an unyielding amount of energy and they often act out inappropriately. Recent studies have also shown us that the central nervous system plays a large role in the functioning of learning and coping skills.

Researchers have also found this condition to be associated with the neurotransmitter deficiency ailment. The neurotransmitter process is associated with the central nervous system and problems then become noticeable. If this can be treated then the disorder may be treated as well because they are linked.

Diet may play a large role in this condition as well. Most patients who are diagnosed often lack in a healthy diet. Parents are advised to contact a professional if their child exhibits these behaviors and they will look at your child's diet with you to ensure they are receiving the proper nutrients for a healthy central nervous system. The patient who is not diagnosed may become suicidal.

ADHD is common in children and many of these children will resort to drugs and alcohol to relieve themselves of their symptoms. If your child is suspected of suffering from this condition then they should receive proper treatment and therapy. You also need to ensure the diet is not deficient in any nutrients as this does have an effect. Many children will require a good diet plan, therapy, natural supplements, and chiropractic tactics.

Impulsive Behaviors

Impulse Control Disorders are becoming more common in today's children. There are few people, who have never acted on an impulse, but when symptoms are reoccurring and consistent then the individual needs help. Judgment plays a large role in impulses and if the judgment is ignored in a dangerous situation someone may get hurt.

Most of the individuals suffering from this condition act on impulses against their better judgment. In many cases these behaviors hurt others. These individuals also tend to not have the ability to regard the law, society, themselves or others. They simply act without thinking. The patient also has an intense feeling to act out on an impulse even though his instinct says "no."

Intermittent Explosive Disorder is the worst of these conditions because the end result can be deadly if left untreated. These individuals illustrate explosive behaviors and patients with this disorder have neurological and brain aberrations. Many of these individuals are very dangerous and other mental illnesses are often lurking beneath the surface. For example, a child could be diagnosed with Intermittent Explosive Disorders, Impulsive Control Disorder, Antisocial Disorder, Oppositional Defiance and Psychopathic Tendencies. These individuals can be hard to treat and many will tell you there is no treatment for them.

These individuals will do several dangerous acts including:

Kevin Green

•Abuse a person to the point of death

•Bash walls

•Bust windows

•Terrorize the home

•Hurt animals

•Start fires

•Make explosives

•Engage in pornographic materials obsessively

•Laugh for no reason

•Walk around with a deranged look

This is also just the beginning of their actions in many ways. These individuals will also show no remorse for their actions and may even blackout during their explosions. These individuals also appear to have a good side and an evil side. They tend to be triggered by certain actions or words, but they may also explode for no apparent reason. Founding counseling for these individuals is often difficult if you can find them at all.

Many will simply tell you that it is hereditary and there is nothing they can do for you. Parents can deal with these children by showing absolutely no fear for them and using reverse psychology. Impulse Control Disorders also include Pathological Gambling Obsessions.

Don't Forget Your Mental Health
This activity is often uncontrollable as well once the addiction of gambling sets in. These people may also have underlying disorders such as:

•Antisocial personalities

•Mood swings

•Alcohol and drug addiction

•Depression

•OCD

These individuals also resort to theft and kleptomania. Pyromaniacs are also placed in this category because they are unable to control their impulses. These individuals set fires and watch them burn. They will also extend this beyond their own home. These people have issues with substance abuse, self-esteem; resist authority and other similar symptoms. If you notice someone sitting around and burning items in the home and laughing about it you will want to watch this person closely. Some individuals only show slight symptoms while others will be more severe.

Chapter 5- Stress-Induced Mental Disorders

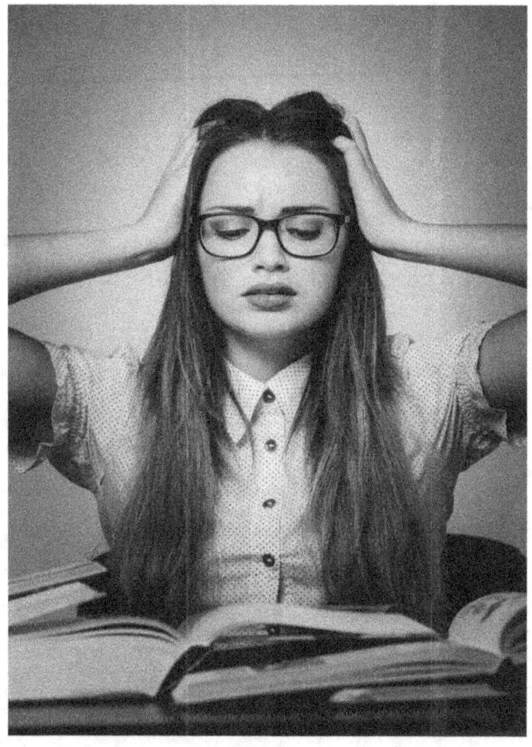

Multiple Personality Disorder and Posttraumatic Stress

These two conditions are often linked together because the person may develop additional personalities to deal with their stress. These patients are often the survivors of severe abuse. Multiple Personality Disorders often have several symptoms including:

•Distinct personalities

•Personalities of different genders

•Personalities of different ages

•Multiple signatures

Don't Forget Your Mental Health
•Different IQs

•Personality Types

•Amnesia

•Voices in the head

•Frequent nightmares

•The use of "we" when referring to self

•Outer body experiences

These patients are often alone in the world because the experts do not usually have enough information to understand their diagnosis. It is often difficult to ever hear the truth about these conditions as well. These patients will often fight against lying and will strive for accuracy. Female patients are rarely violent, while males may be. Some males patients have been sent to prison for crimes including robbery and rape. Patients often act on projection or interjection caused by an alter personality.

This condition has been questioned as whether or not it is real, but the fact is that it is a true condition. Many have tried to pretend to have multiple personalities to get out of crimes by way of insanity, but it is nearly impossible for these individuals to maintain distinct personalities. Personalities may include child alters, teens, adults and even elderly personalities. All personalities are a sub part of the actual person who has been traumatized to the point that they are no longer able to cope.

These individuals are also very intelligent. These individuals tend to have issues and difficulty with medical treatment as their blood pressure may raise and lower, they may have seizures and their respiratory rates may change. Some personalities may even be blind. The patient often goes through life with the disorder and when they reach a certain age they have no chance of coping. This is when integration of the personalities needs to occur. Integration places the alter personalities in an area of the mind to stay permanently.

Once the integration is complete, these individuals may have a hard time going back to normal life as they have lived most of their life with their "family" in their mind. These individuals have a sense of loss because they don't know how to cope in the world without their personalities. It is possible for the personalities to communicate with each other after integration, but it is never the same. Many individuals have a difficult time going through life because they are used to the daily stress of work and life being shared by their other personalities and now they only have themselves to depend on.

Underdeveloped Child Separation

Many emotional breakdowns are caused by individuals who have not separated from their inner person at childhood. Many mental illnesses in society are complicated because we do not always see to the root of the problem. The child within exists throughout our lifetime and if we do not recognize this "inner child" we tend to suffer from emotional breakdowns. As a result, many professionals struggle to find a way to treat patients with this disorder.

Many of these people were ignored as children and were emotionally neglected and maybe even physically abuse and many have witnessed bad scenes in life that haunt them. Unless the problems are dealt with the issue continues to grow. To contact the inner self the person has to have a basic knowledge of their problem. Once a basic knowledge is situation, the person is then able to move on to the next step. Once a person has basic understanding of themselves they are able to move forward with the help of therapy.

Many diagnoses stem from brain injuries, chemical and physical imbalances. Effective treatment is not always possible until the person is able to deal with their problems. For example, a schizophrenic was once found to have a disease of the mind because the twin holes of the brain had a larger side to the cavity of the brain. This condition is also genetic and many of these people have disruptive childhoods and will often deny that happenings occurred.

As long as the patient is in denial, it is difficult to impossible to treat them. Another example can also be seen when patients are diagnosed with posttraumatic stress disorder. These patients were also subjected to trauma in their childhood and the disorder escalates during that experience. The solution for this is to address the child beneath the disorder and then move forward to treat the trigger of the disorder. Once you dig deep enough you will be able to help the patient become acquainted with the child within and then treat the patient more effectively.

Many people have difficulty treating these disorders because they do not completely listen to the patient. Many therapists have the idea of they are holding the degree so they know more than the patient does. If more people listened then this would not be such an issue in society. The best solution begins with listening to the patient and actually hearing what they are saying. These individuals often have to take things one day at a time as well.

CHAPTER 6- PERSONALITY DISORDERS

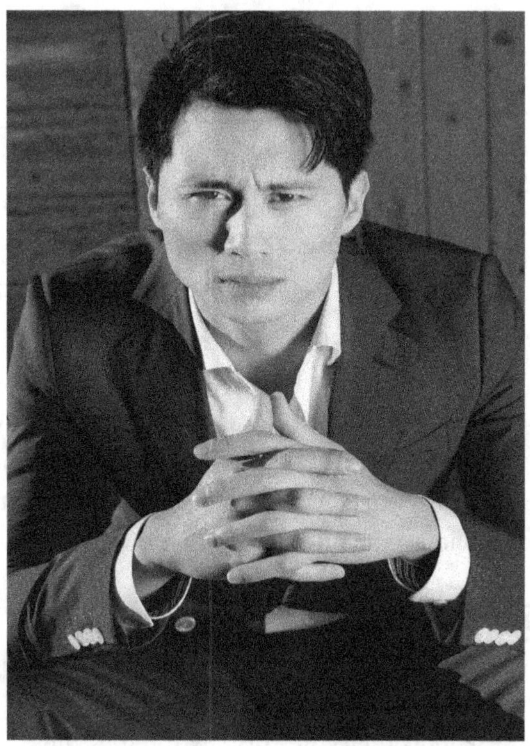

There are several types of personality disorders. Some we have already discussed and others we have mentioned. Now we talk about the various other disorders that have been alluded to and are often combined with other mental illnesses.

Borderline Personality Disorder

Borderline Personality Disorder symptoms include:

•Impulsive behaviors

•Unpredictable mood swings

•Terrified of being abandoned

•Promiscuous behaviors

•Manipulation

•Self-destructive behavior

•Violence behavior

It is possible to treat these individuals but they can be dangerous to live with. These individuals may cut themselves to seek attention and may even threaten suicide. They tend to offer a love/hate relationship and will seek similar characteristics in other individuals. Other symptoms may include short-term psychotic breaks, illicit behaviors, depression, demanding behaviors and denial. This disorder is linked to incest, emotional breakdowns in families and alcoholism and drug addiction.

Histrionic Personality Types

These types often act and will play the role of the victim in most situations. These individuals may display the following:

•Vanity

•Narcissism

•Anger

•Seductive

•Flirty

•Extreme violence to the point of murder

These individuals may be diagnosed with other illnesses as well.

Obsessive Compulsive Disorders

These conditions are known by their behaviors. These people tend to display the following:

•Disregard for rules and regulations

•Perfectionists

•Inability to complete tasks

•Controlling with one type of person, such as less authority figures

•Acts out of self-control around authority figures to hid their identity

•Views people as objects

This type is common and is often domestically violent individuals. These individuals often have the problem of completing tasks because they are not very flexible people and disregard other feelings and emotions. These patients tend to abuse others that show emotion to them. All of the personality types listed above tends to have a look of seriousness at all times. They may force themselves to laugh around others.

All of these personality types tend to be dangerous as they do not have any feelings for others. Many of the individuals who commit homicides suffer from one of the following:

•Antisocial Personality Disorder

•Borderline Personality Disorder

•Histrionic Personality Disorder

•OCD – it is reported that these individuals kill slowly

•Psychopathic

•Sociopath

•Schizophrenia

These individuals are difficult to treat and in some cases impossible if the person refuses to accept help.

Passive Aggressive Disorders

Passive-Aggressive Personality types often sabotage various areas of their life in the sense that they complain about demands that are put on them. They may not voice their complaints but they are cussing them out in their minds and the person or thing that made them do the work.

Passive-Aggressive types are exactly as the name implies. They are often passive outwards, but aggressive inwards. These people often anger others around them, yet the person may feel wrong for not being clear on the foundation that caused the anger. These types of people are also deceiving as they use obscure tactics in persecuting others.

For example, say Troy confronts Kelly expressing to him that her behaviors were wrong and that they were causing problems. Kelly looks at Troy with a glare tells Kelly that he is the problem. Kelly says she did what she was supposed to and that he did nothing wrong that Troy doesn't know what he's talking about.

This disorder often causes controversy and is often disputed, but the term is used frequently. Self-Defeating Personality Disorders often associate with person that will cause harm to persecute the person or self-defeat them. This person will also excuse another person's offer to help them even if the help is needed. This type of person may also anger others around them and then display hurt when they are confronted.

These two personality types are not able to hold permanent relationships in most cases and will make excuses for their behavior. Sadistic Personality Disorders were recently removed from the DSM manual because of a lack of foundation for diagnosis. The symptoms included not being able to control their behavior. These people are violent and will harm others to uphold control over another person.

This disorder is similar to psychopathic and antisocial personality disorders and may rejoice when they hurt other people or animals. Even if the person is submissive, the person will often torture or hurt others because it gives them pleasure. Persons that suffer from this disorder are often survivors of abuse and are angry at the world around them. These individuals cannot typically maintain a relationship and will hurt the person involved in their life.

Chapter 7- How Stress Affects Your Mental Health

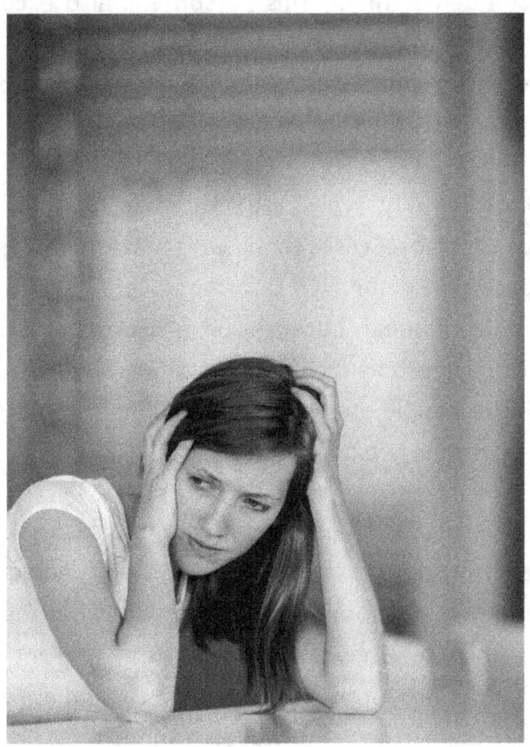

Stress and how it affects the mental health of a person is not something to take lightly. It can impact the mental health of a person in more ways than one.

Stress has positive and negative effects. For the positive side, stress can make a person system surge and jump up to be more productive; enabling a person to meet impossible deadlines and letting you finish tasks that you thought were impossible.

On the negative side, stress can inhibit a person from really functioning. More often than not, it limits a person's thinking or reasoning; it can hold someone back and slows them down from accomplishing the tasks that they need to do. Stress acts like a stop sign that freezes a person in his tracks.

What Can Stress Do to You

When a person says that he or she is stressed, more often than not, this refers to the negative form of stress. The mind and body feels the tension that stress is in putting on the system. There are instances where stress and its effects are short lived and whatever impact they may have on the system are minimal to none.

Then there occasions where stress is long term, and the effects are often long lasting and majorly impacts the system, both mentally and physically.

There are many ailments and diseases that are related to stress. Understand that stress affects the whole body. From the major organs like the heart, lungs, kidneys and then you also have the brain. Physically and mentally when a person is overloaded or stretched beyond his or her limit, just like a rubber band, the body as a whole feels the effects.

One example of a stress related ailment is depression. If you define depression, it means that a person is suffering from a low mood and at times he or she has an aversion for activities. It also affects the behavior, thoughts and feelings of a person. It is manifested in feelings like hopelessness, despair, lack of vigor, feeling of loss and restlessness.

A person who is depressed lacks the vitality that he or she once felt. Depression also affects concentration, often making the person forgetful. It can also affect the appetite of the person suffering from depression, thus manifesting in loss of energy, fatigue, aches and pains and at times digestive problems.

Depression and Mental Health

When you really think about it, depression which is caused by stress will target a person's mental health and over all wellbeing. The mood in itself is not a psychiatric disorder, since it is a normal reaction of the mind to the events that are happening in life. But as it progresses, this stress related disorder can become something serious.

There have been many cases where people who suffer from depression are often treated with medicine since whatever they are feeling is starting to affect their health, mentally and physically and their safety. Just like with people who are suicidal or for those who become dependent and abuse drugs.

How to Avoid Stress-Induced Disorders

You need to remember that when you are going through a situation that is stressful, you need to find ways to relieve it. How would vary from person to person. There are many ways and outlets where you can ease impact of stress in your life.

Suggested Ways:

Exercise – remember that when you exercise, you are enabling the body to produce endorphins, often called the happy hormones. These hormones are produced by the pituitary gland and the hypothalamus and they act like drug in your system, easing the pain and tension that you feel in your body and produces an overall sense of wellbeing.

Sleep – this is one of the most basic ways on how a person can get some relief from stress. Sleep is important since it helps the mind and body to regenerate and relax. Remember that when you are facing a stressful situation, your mind is on overload. You are triggering your body to produce an overload of hormones that in most cases, will lead to harming your system. When you sleep, you are letting your body and mind to take its much needed rest. You are helping your system to shut down and cool off.

Have you ever noticed that when you have a good night's sleep, you just feel recharged, alert and ready to face the day? This is how sleep helps you to relieve stress

Meditation – another alternative that you can use is to do practice meditation. Meditation is actually letting your mind relax and achieve state of calmness while you are awake. It's like stepping into a place where you can find peace and happiness, detaching yourself from the world and all the stress that you will ever feel. It promotes relaxation, it lets you build internal energy, enhance your concentration, and overall achieve a sense of well-being.

Pampering – for some, they find ways to relieve stress through leisure. It can be in the form of shopping, going to the spa and getting a massage or going to the salon, getting manis and pedis or getting their hair done. Pampering is one form of leisure that is a sure fire way of relieving stress.

Travelling – another of leisurely activities that many people opt for when they want to relieve stress. In a way, this is a form of detachment from the situation or place where they feel the tension. Being able to escape and relax the mind often helps people to ease the stress that they are feeling in the system.

Last on the list...

Talking – one of the most basic, primary and easiest way to relieve stress. When you are undergoing something that is putting a strain in your system, or when you have a problem, or when you just feel that you are being pulled from all sides and you are about to break, what you need to do is just sit back and talk to someone about the situation.

Talking is a cure all, since it releases tension from your body and it enables you to analyze the situation that you are going through. When you talk to someone whom you can trust, you are able to release the negative emotions that are stored inside you. By talking about the situation, you are now helping your body and mind to release the stress that is stored inside.

CHAPTER 8- HEALING COMES FROM YOUR SPIRITUAL SELF

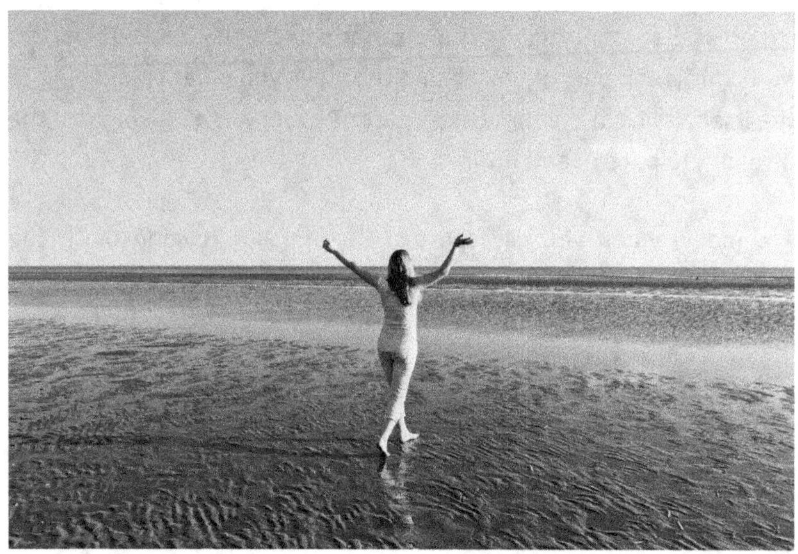

When you say spiritual health, what does it really pertain to? In addressing the overall wellness of a person, there are three essential components, comprising of the mental, physical and Spiritual health.

When you really analyze it, spiritual health is the most important part of the overall wellbeing of a person. Aside from the mental and physical aspects of life that we take into account, spiritual wellness is an essential factor for health.

Have you ever noticed happy people and why they rarely get sick? What is the answer to this? Well, this person is healthy spiritually.

Understanding Spiritual Health

Spiritual Health pertains to a person emotional wellbeing and wholeness. If a person is spiritually imbalanced, then mental and physical they will also feel imbalanced. There is a deep and intertwined connection between our emotions, our mind and our body. If a person is feeling spiritually healthy, the mind would feel more alert and the body will also feel healthy and fit.

When you say spiritual, you are pertaining to the deepest part of you. This is the part of your being that tells you what is meaning of life itself. It lies in the innermost part of your system, giving you the strength to believe and hope.

For many, when you say spiritual, it refers to religion or to the connection to God. For others, it is the emotions that are inside, or the personal relationships that they have with others.

Addressing Your Spiritual Health

Remember that there is a great and deep connection between your mental, physical and spiritual aspects. All of these play an important role when it comes to your health.

Spiritual wellness and health takes the back burner, which really shouldn't be the case. When a person is spiritually healthy, the body and mind follows. If a person is dissatisfied, unhappy, experiences feelings of emptiness, then that person's spiritual health is suffering.

The effect of this to the system is that the body feels fatigued, often stressed out, and the mind does not function as it should be, and you often lose your concentration or you lose your focus and drive to finish your tasks.

When you feel well and balanced spiritually, you will have an overall sense of wellbeing. This is as important as the food, water and knowledge that you feed your system. Being healthy spiritually will give you the comfort that you need, enlighten you with the purpose for the things that you need to do, give you the strength that you need and then there is hope and inner peace.

You need to address your spiritual health because this is the fuel keeps a person to go on. This is where the inner strength of a person lies, and if this part is not healthy, you will not have that drive to keep you in motion.

Determination, strength, faith, hope, ambition, purpose – these are just some of the many gifts that our spiritual health offers us.

How to Help Yourself Spiritually

How do you help yourself spiritually and how do you make it healthy? Tough question? Not really.

When you really look at it, there are many ways on how you can keep yourself spiritually healthy. Again and again, it all starts with you.

Discovering Spiritual Wellness

Maintaining spiritual wellness is a conscious act that a person should take into account. Connecting to the core, to that essential life force that is ingrained in you is the key in answering and maintaining your spiritual health.

Spiritual health in not just about religion, though it is part of it. The reality is that spiritual health comes before religion, since this is what connects us to our faith and our beliefs.

Spirituality is actually the connection that we have with the meaning and purpose that you have in life. It is the discovery of who you are and what you can do. It is the balance that provides you with inner strength, with hope and with inner peace.

Be Still and Listen

When you tune in to your inner voice and you really identify the factors that make you whole, you are feeding your spirit and helping it to grow. In meditation practices like yoga and breathing exercises, you are channeling your mind and body and letting the spirit grow and take precedence.

It is important that we should feed and nourish the spiritual side of our lives. By taking simple walks, letting all of the stress go, prayer, finding peace and harmony, you are giving food to your spirit.

Remember that you should never neglect your spiritual health. There are many people who are really aware of this side of life. A lot of people are bitter, angry, lonely, skeptical and violent because they forgot to nourish their spirit and just let it deteriorate. They feel embittered of life and they feel that they do not have the will or purpose to survive each day. If you really think about it, you would ask what happened to them.

These types of people who are just lacking when it comes to the drive and the will to survive forgot to stay connected to what is essential. They let the daily machinations of life take over and they forgot to feed the most important part of their being.

Self Help

Stay connected to what really defines you. Find ways to enrich your spiritual side. There are many ways, and all of them will need you to act as the person and the instigator. Remember that there is no force on earth that can make you move if you do not want to move. You need to be aware of what you need and what will work for you.

For many religion and the connection to the divine is the food that they need. For some it is the connection to nature that nourished their spirit. Then there are others who find fulfillment in helping others. Find your niche and stay there or you can combine and mix and match to enrich and feed you spirit to make it healthy.

CHAPTER 9- LETTING GO OF THE ILL-EFFECTS OF ANGER AND GRIEF

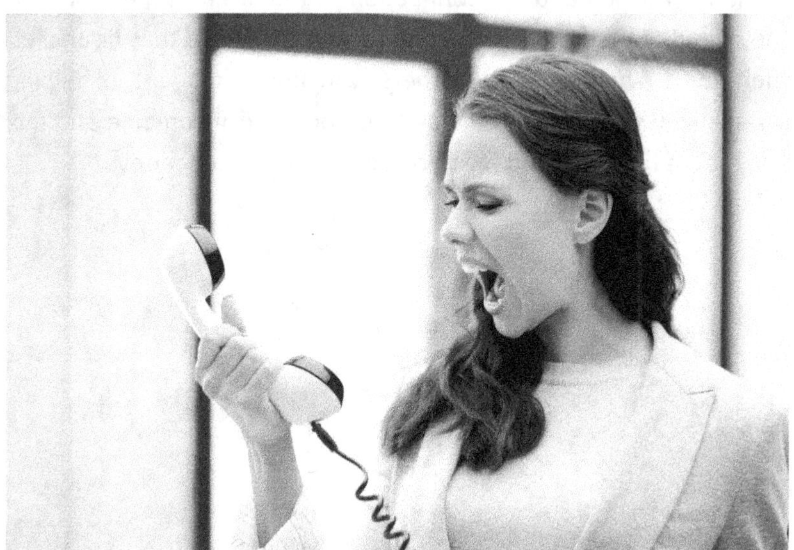

Have you ever noticed how the body reacts when you are angry? The reaction would be that the body heats up, and then there are times when your hands and body shake, and you have this uncontrollable urge to do something physical.

What about when you experience grief? And what about when have that feeling of loss and despair? How does your body react? What is the effect in the system?

These are some points to consider when you are dealing with anger and grief and how does it impact you overall health, mentally and physically.

What is Anger?

Anger is an emotion that is tied up with strong uncomfortable responses due to a provocation. It is the psychological interpretation of the system when it is offended, denied or wronged. External expressions of anger would be change in facial expression or body language, and some cases, acts of aggression.

What is Grief?

Grief is the response of the system to loss. To be particular, this is the loss of someone who is important to a person. Though primarily focused on the emotional response of the body, there are also reactions from the physical, behavioral, social, cognitive and philosophical aspects of the system. External expressions of grief would be crying, hysteria and in severe cases would be loss of consciousness.

Reaction to Anger and Grief

Anger and grief are powerful emotions. When a person is angry, the physical reactions would be that of an increased heart rate, surges in the levels of adrenaline, and an increase in blood pressure. Anger is a predominant feeling when it comes to the cognitive, behavioral and psychological makeup of a person. As for grief, pertaining to loss, the reaction of the body is shock.

Both of these intense emotions play a great havoc in the system. These are manifested in the biological, emotional and mental reactions of the body which releases something that affects the physiological and neurological processes.

The Impact

When a person experiences grief or anger, the impact that it brings to the system is really big. Since these are strong emotions, the effects that they have are also powerful.

Don't Forget Your Mental Health

When a person experiences grief and feelings of loss, depression is really just around the corner. Then there is the have loss of appetite which leads to drastic weight loss, hair loss, dry skin, digestive problems, mental anguish, lack of concentration and more. For anger, there are effects like high blood pressure which may lead to heart attack and damages to the arteries because of the increased heart rate that a person experiences.

When you really look at it, anger and grief, along with other emotions play an important part in a person's wellbeing. Unless properly address, these feelings of anger and grief will control and may destroy a person mentally as well as physically. The overall impact cannot be really gauged because the tolerance of the body for these types of emotions varies from person to person.

How do You Help Yourself Get Rid of Anger and Grief?

In relieving your mind and body with the stress of anger and grief, you need to look for outlets as a way of self-help.

Just like with any problem, you need to deal with the issues that you have.

For anger, since this aggression, you can divert it. You can channel your energy and burn out your anger through exercise. For some people, they opt to divert their attention and anger to doing something that is productive or something that will calm them.

There are many productive ways where you can help yourself in handling your aggression. You do not need to become violent and abusive; instead you can make it productive.

For grief and loss, understand that you need to go through the process. You need to go through shock and denial, then you have intense concern, where you are not able to think of anything else, then you have despair and depression and then at last to recovery.

For the first three stages, you need to make that conscious effort to pull yourself together and go through that stage. While going through these phases, you can enlist the help of someone that is close to you to watch over you so that you do not go over the deep end.

Remember that even in the midst of pain and loss, you can still make a conscious effort that you will not be in one stage of the process and get stuck there.

Self Help

There are many self-help books and motivational materials out there telling people of what they can do and how they can do it when it comes to overcoming grief and anger. The real secret behind these books is the word self-help.

You need to help yourself in order to recover. Just like a wound, you cannot just leave it alone and not clean it. If you do not clean your wound, it would fester and it would cause you more harm and more damage. You do not really want that to happen do you?

When you are through anger and grief, always remember that the only person that could help you is you. Sure there are people that you can go to in seeking help like shrinks and doctors to help you medically or you go spiritual counselors who will give you advice and counseling. But at the end of the day, all you need is you.

The struggle and the battle will always begin and end within you. Since you have the power to overcome these emotions, pull

Don't Forget Your Mental Health
yourself together, reflect on the situation and decide to get out of the clutches of these damaging emotions.

Remember that if you do not deal with your anger or your grief, you are not just hurting the people around you, you are harming yourself. You are damaging your system, by being stuck with anger and rage, or you are destroying your system by being depressed with grief and loss.

CHAPTER 10- HOW TO RELATE TO PEOPLE WITH MENTAL ILLNESS

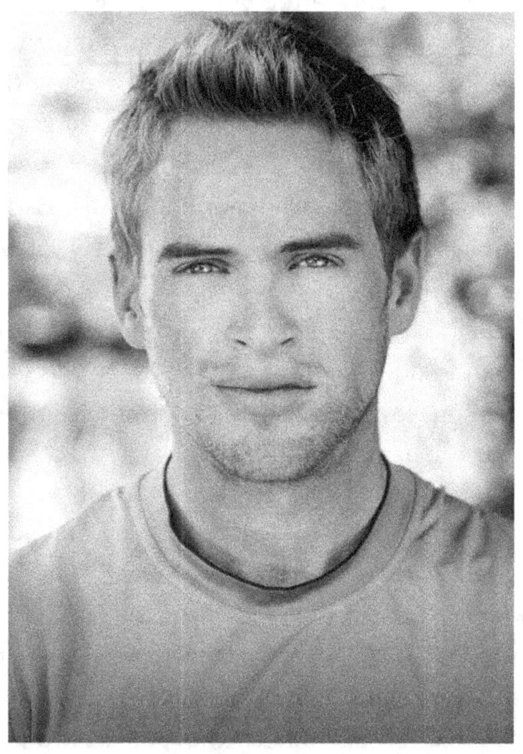

Relating to others with disabilities is often difficult. If you have a mental illness the only sources that understand you most times in the mental health experts, and sometimes they fail. I cannot count on 90 peoples' finger and toes how many patients told me that mental health experts were not helping them. The patients were complaining about the medications and treatment they were receiving. The problem may have lain between the patient and therapist, since sometimes patients do not do their best to listen and follow instructions. Other times therapist does not do their best to listen and hear, what the patient is telling them. Regardless, something is not working, so we need to learn effective strategies that help us to relate to disabilities. Often when a patient is complaining there is a source that lead to that complaint.

In some cases were the diagnosis is affected by pretense (certain disorders cause patients to complain even if there are not a problem), while most disabilities there is a source and reason for the complaint. Here is part of the problem. When the person has a source of complaint, they are often ignored simply because they have a mental illness. You are exaggerating is often the sentence used when a mental ill patient complains. In most cases this is not true, since mental ill patients are often more aware of their surroundings than the so-called normal minds. Schizophrenias, psychotics, drug-induced disorders, and a few other types of mental illnesses include symptoms of hallucination, voices, delusions and illusions. The patients will complain that their voices are telling them to do something, and although this is a degree of pretense or misunderstanding, it is important to listen since the patient is subject to harm him or herself as well as others around.

When a person has a delusional state of mind and voices outside the head, then there is no room for disregarding the patient. However, when a patient does not have symptoms listed above they often are vigilant, and can explain what is happening to them. One other problem is the therapist or others around the patient will often attempt to disconnect the patient from his or her complaint. In other words, they will tell the patient what the problem is, and avoid hearing what the patient is telling them.

Reading between the lines is the best solution for communication and understanding, however most people read between their own lines when communicating. I cannot stress the disadvantages this action causes, since communication is vital for humans to get along and understand one another. Dialect often plays a role in failure of communication, since we are all different and few of us can understand dialect. Therefore, one effective method of communicating and relating to disabilities is to grasp hold of dialect and learn how to read between the lines of the patients. It is important to continue consistent understanding strategies to help the patient cope with his or her symptoms. Another great strategy is "Role-Play."

Role Play is great since the patient can look inside his or her self through a separate pair of eyes while examining the cause and action of the problem. Stepping outside of your own mind helps you to see between the lines, and helps the patient to grasp hold of the solution in front of them. For example, the patient may be living a harmful lifestyle that triggers their symptoms and is unaware of their actions and behaviors. If the patient includes all elements of the problem in the picture and views it with an open mind or another eye, then the patient will most likely see the cause of their problem. This method is also effective for helping the patient see who was a part of their symptoms, such as the person may have been abused which caused the persons symptoms to a degree. If that person comes to accept the problem then that patient can move forward in life successfully.

Acceptance then is the other issue we must address to learn, and relate to disabilities, as well as relate to everyone around us. Understanding mental illness can help us to find the answers to the many problems around us.

Giving the Mentally Ill the Gift of Understanding

Understanding mental illness can help us help loved ones recover from their suffering. Although it is not possible to completely understand since even scientist is often baffled, it is possible to have a basic understanding. Understanding mental health and trauma can also help us to learn more about mental illnesses. The problem starts at the door with the mental health experts. They often start out diagnosing the patient upfront, and lay out a series of diagnosis that will cover medical cost on insurance.

The next step is finding the diagnosis that insurance will cover if long-term treatment is needed. As you can see upfront that, the patient is already headed for additional problems, since money is the primary issue when it comes to mental health. The patient is the last to know in many cases that he or she just stepped into a web of financial issues and entrapment treatment. In other words the patient could be diagnosed with Axis 1: Depression: Axis II: Bipolar: Axis III: Physical problems: Axis IV: Psychotic Episodes: Axis V: suicidal with serious interrupted symptoms surrounding the cause.

This is obviously a serious complaint and insurance will often consider coverage since the patient is a hazard. After they are interview by an intake therapist, they are often shifted to the next level, therapy. After the therapist evaluates the patient sorting through the intakes information and watching the patient for signs or traces of symptoms related, the next level the therapist uses is diagnosing the patient with a mental disorder that complies with coverage.

Most patients are diagnosed properly however, few are incorrectly diagnosed. The next level is visiting the psychiatrist who will then administer medications to treat the patient; since more money is involved they must understand what Medicaid or other insurance policies will cover. The patient is then subject to a therapist and a psychiatrist that believes they know more than the patient does. In regards to psychological disadvantages this is true, however if the patient was willing to do some research he or she might have more an advantage over the professionals since they are informed. Once they understand what symptoms are in the different diagnosis, they can then help the counselor and doctor understand more about their suffering.

Kevin Green
The best solution then is to research the diagnosis that the therapist placed on you to see if this is what you are going through. Study the symptoms carefully weeding out any elements of the diagnosis that may not involve you. After you have weeded through the rumble, the next step is sitting down with your therapist and letting them know that you took steps in your own recovery. You have evaluated the many diagnoses, including the diagnoses the therapist issued, and found that there are elements missing or there are elements of the diagnose that was overwrought. After you discuss with your therapist the potentials or the elements of the diagnose that was misunderstood you both can then work toward reaching an overall view of what is really go on in your life.

It is important that you take notes if you have difficulty staying focused, or if you lack education, you might want to get a love one to help you with the research, notes and discussing the problem with your therapist. When we know what is going on, and what we are dealing with inside...This is a part of understanding the problem and how it connects to the people around you is if you understand what is going on within your mind, and then you can explain this to your friends and loved ones, helping them to understand. After we see where the problem lies we can then move onto the next step and start accepting that there is a problem.

Dealing with the problems is your next step, which takes understanding. If you do not have understanding then the problem will only regress. Tell your loved ones and friends that you are working toward treatment and it would be helpful if they too work with you to help you find a recovery in your mental health problems. If there is no recovery, then they can work with you, understanding that you will have symptoms erupt from time to time and they will know which step to take to helping you cope.

Yet, we must look at entertainment and how it plays a role in mental health issues.

How Entertainment Helps

Ironically, studies have shown that certain types of movies, music and reading materials are linked to mental illnesses. For example, pornographic material has been proven to affect individuals dramatically to the point of murder, rape and other violent crimes. Such materials affect even an individual without mental illnesses simply because someone falls victim to a predator along the path. Violent movies and music has also proven to affect the mind. More and more children today are violent, and studies have shown that video games, movies and music play a large role in the children's behaviors.

Studies has also shown that children are committing murder, rape, taking drugs, alcohol, and interrupting others peoples life as a result from obsessive entertainment behaviors. Although few argue that this is ludicrous, they have no idea what they are talking about, since the ones arguing are the sources that are producing such interrupting noises. Not so long ago a young man claimed after hearing the song "Kill your Mother" countless of times, the lyrics went to his head and he acted out accordingly to the song. This is only one account linked to entertainment and mental health.

Mental health is nothing to toy with and the rules were laid out from the beginning. Even God acknowledged and made it aware to everyone that such behaviors would cause disaster. Proven faithful to His words, the word is going mad because of polluted behaviors created by entertainment. Do not get me wrong, not all entertainment is bad. However, the truth is if you are associating with bad, then bad will come to you and everyone around you because of the action. However, if you are associating with good, then rewards are sure to follow. Not everyone with mental illnesses however engage in wrongful behaviors, actions, or self-exposing themselves to entertainment that harms. At least not directly, but somewhere in their lifetime they were exposed indirectly to this type of behavior. I am promising you that everyone in their lifetime has been exposed to this behavior, everyone with the exceptions of newborns. It is time we look at what goes on around us to improve mental health. We will be pounding our heads against the walls for a lifetime if we do not admit that harmful entertainment is part of the problem.

Children learn what they hear, see, and are taught. Likewise, adults learn what they see, hear and are taught. No one is an exception the rule, and all of us are subjects to influences. Life is too short to be playing around with dangers. Either we are in this together are we are all working toward a disastrous future. Satisfaction guaranteed since it is showing in all areas of life. Take the terrorist attack in New York recently. What do you think linked this mental ailment to reality? While there are many explanations and reasons, the main reason is the culprits were exposed to violence during their lifetime and this is what they knew according to what they saw, worked. In addition, it did to a degree.

Somewhere down the line people were communicating, however very few were listening, otherwise this would not have happen in the first place. Somebody in this picture was complaining and trying to express their emotions and thoughts, yet somebody on the other side was ignoring the cries. What it boils down to is how a person believes. If a person believes after being taught that violence is the answer to resolve a problem, then violence is what you are going to see and everyone will be affected as a result. You do not play around with faith, either you are in the race to win, or else you are on the road to death.

Finally, we can see that entertainment is today more graphic, and depicts inexplicit pictures on nearly every channel, radio station, and so on today. It seems the morals and values are going down the tube, while the world is going deeper and deeper into chaos and war. No one can fix a problem as quickly as the problem occurred, but somewhere someone has to get started to resolving what has already been done. How do ill minds think alike?

Do Ill Minds Really Think Alike?

Some people believe that mental illnesses are all the same. If you are diagnosed with a mental illness then not to worry because everyone else diagnosed is just like you. This is far removed from reality and the truth. What is so ironic is the same people that are saying this (is often ill them self) will often say something to the affect when a murder takes place. 'He is a psychopathic or sociopath. Yet the neighbor down the road who visits every day has a mental illness and when this person visits, or the therapist is overwrought.

You do not have a mental illness you have problems like the rest of us. This is easier to accept than believing that a person has a mental illness. This is nuts, since it is only contributing to the problem. The problem with the world is all the people seeking help are doing their job and the people that are making excuses or in denial of mental health, illness existence is in serious need of help. For example if Johnny visits a counselor knowing that something is not right, he is asking for help.

On the other hand if that person sitting at the table telling the neighbor nothing is wrong, and claims that seeing a counselor is only spending money, then guess who is in real need of help. The person that does not go to a counselor or ask someone in the world for help is the person that mentally ill more so than the common mental ill. Mental is nothing to play around with, and since we are all different it can be complicated to determine who is ill. I have watched as countless of patients went to mental health experts and watched them continue to suffer although they worked hard with the counselor to find a resolve. The problem is that mental health experts are more concerned about money than the patients are most time, and believe they know it all and the patient knows nothing most all the time.

Many therapists are in this field of expertise and if you did a background check on the professional, you are probably going to see this person is a mental health potential or skip out as well. It does not take a genius to understand mental health, but it takes many idiots to tangle the webs of darkness. In most instances, mentally ill patients are brilliant individuals that have difficulty managing their lives due to frequent interruptions. Most all the patients that go to mental health experts can talk about their problems freely searching for answers to survive.

The problem is (between the lines of communication) lies a fountain of information that can help both the patient and the counselor, but too many times the counselors are entangled in their own webs, they miss out on the benefits of helping another person out. Personally, I spent 25 years in counselor with no results up until the last three years and then I was working harder than the counselor to resolve my own problems was. She was doing a portion of her job, but my strategies were succeeding hers, and I left her behind. Now, if you see what I am saying then you will know that anyone with a mental illness has more of an answer than over half of the professionals in the world. If you have, experience and they have a piece of paper without experience, who knows more? I often have more compassion for mentally ill patients, than I have for the so-called normal and professionals of the world. I have watched many suffering after begging practically for help, and very little result came from it all. I watched as many counselors blamed the patient for the failure, but in all truths, they had a responsibility in this as well.

Most counselors are in denial which is a mental health issue, and many people in many professions are in denial, and this my friend is a major cause for mental health issues around the world. Ill minds think alike because someone is influenced while the other source is influencing. A great source for learning and understanding is group therapy.

The Effectivity of Group Therapy

Group therapy has proven to be effective in mental health. While some counselor will start out with one on one therapy, they may finally refer the patient to group sessions. Many services and support groups available offer help to those with mental health problems. Group therapy allows the patients to freely discuss their issues, problems, and even find social influences that share the same symptoms or similar symptoms. When two or more people can relate to each other, this is often more effective than one-on-one sessions.

Group therapy sessions allow the patients to meet once or twice each week, meeting many others that share common illnesses, thus promoting association. If a person is suffering and has difficult to meet in public places, or even go grocery shopping this is a great source for healing. Some people with mental illnesses often avoid socializing simply because they feel that other people do not understand and it is embarrassing for them to go in public when they are at risk of erupting from their diagnose.

Triggers are often what cause a mental ill individual to suffer interruptions, and many times people care less about what may trigger another individual. It is important to get help when you have a mental illness, yet it is also important to work through the problems on your own if possible. If you use self-talk strategies, it can help with your mental health issues. Another great form of therapy is writing your problems on paper. This is great since if you put all the details of your interruptions on paper your counselor can help you find out the cause and work toward a resolve. Other great strategy for dealing with mental health is to avoid isolation. This is where group therapy comes in to play. Since you are around others, you will be able to communicate.

Communication is an excellent source for healing. Another great source for healing is education. If you are in a group therapy session, you are teaching more about you disability as well as learning about how others suffer similar symptoms as yourself. This prevents you from feeling alone. Group therapy is also great since it gives you the ability to get out of the house. Think of it as an activity or a social entertaining experience. The entertainment will be seen once you sit down, relax and start sharing your problems with others. Most people when you tell them I am suffering from my diagnosis, symptoms including the inability to concentrate; most people will say, 'oh, I understand this. I too have difficulties concentrating.' Well, what do you do to make matters better? You may ask. The other person may tell you what he or she does to work toward concentrating, and you may see somewhere in the conversation a strategy that can work for you. It becomes entertainment since you found a source of happiness within.

Group therapy is great for many individuals, but there are some disorders where group therapy should be avoided at all costs. Although counselors have set up group meetings for such disabilities, it often proves troublesome rather than helpful. One example is MPD patients, or Multiple Personality Disorder. These patients are very distinct and have triggers that interrupt the diagnose more so than other types of mental illnesses. Mental illness is tricky and often difficult to understand, but in most all cases, there is a solution to dealing with the diagnoses. It is important to pay close attention if you are joining a group session. When you pay attention, you receive the benefits of hearing all about others and how they suffer too. You also get the benefit of possible learning something about yourself. When you learn who you are, you are growing to development, which is the element required for better mental health.

Finally, many that suffer mental illnesses often lack development. There was something in their lifetime that was not provided to them to help them grow. If a person is now growing in accordance to human standards, then that person often jumps track somewhere along the way. Mental health and group sessions then, is a great solution for growing. Education in mental health is another great source for understanding mental health.

The Role of the Education System in Helping the Mentally Ill

When a person is suffering from mental health issues, then the best source of support and help is found in the educational system. Many people that suffer from mental illness are often in the stone ages and do not realize what is available to them. They were often misinformed while growing up, and since education is always advancing and changing, it is helpful to know what is going on. Of course, if you have a mental illness you will need to see a therapist. However if you are learning this increases your chances of finding hope and avoid being misinformed by someone that is not qualified, or under qualified.

Professionals around the world are constantly searching for answers to the many problems we face today in mental health. The problem is everyone has an answer and most times no one agrees.

They may find an answer to the problem, turn around, and slaughter by analyzing the source to death. Then we have another problem, simply because we have dozens of diagnosis, including schizophrenia, bipolar, depression, trauma, a variety of disorders and so forth. The different diagnoses are diseases of the mind, disorders of the mind, and or chemical and biological interruptions.

To get help we must know what we are dealing with, rather than trusting in others to tell us what is wrong. If we seek out information regarding mental health we might even find an answer to our own problem. We can then inform the professional and assist them with finding a solution to the many problems we face. Mental health is complicated simply because we are dealing with the mind. The mind is tricky and leaves us know room for playing around with illness.

Counseling is nothing more than a common sense strategy laced with education. The professionals are learning constantly new understandings while applying them to the older versions. Somewhere in the middle is an answer and it is often overlooked when a professional will treat several patients during a week and sometimes try to treat each person the same if they have the same diagnose. This is a problem area since are all different in our way, including people with mental illnesses. For example, a counselor may treat two individuals both with schizophrenia.

The counselor may use the same tactics with both patients and medications for treating the patient. One patient may find results and the other patient may complain that the treatment is not working. Why is this happening? Well, it is obvious that one patient may have a different level of schizophrenia, and a different background. Some medications work well with one patient while it may not work at all or work minimal with other patients. The solution then is reevaluating the problem and going over the steps taking to treat the patient and modifying them according to the patients' needs. It is important to recognize a problem to find a method suitable for treating the problem. It is also important to reconcile with the source within.

Meaning if a patient has guilt it is probably because he or she did something that may or may have not been wrong. For example, if a parent taught the child that visiting their friends is wrong (Schizophrenias will often discourage a child from going to other people's home due to the paranoid) and the patient (behind the parents back) went to visit a friend. The patient obviously needs to recognize that he or she did nothing wrong, rather he or she needs to reconcile with self. In this case, the patient will also need to be re-taught to learn right and wrong.

The patient needs to find a resolve. After you have helped the patient overcome this option, it is best to re-teach with material rather than words. Simply put, if the patient has a varied of resources to choose from he or she has the ability to come to their own understanding of what is right or what is wrong. Education is essential for reproving, reforming and instructing a person to the right course in life. Words are also important, since if you do not understand what is said, it is often because of lack of education. Yet we still need to look at the practices in mental health to understand what works best.

About the Author

Kevin Green was born to a dysfunctional family. His mother had problems with alcohol while his dad was almost always never seen around the house. When he was 5 years old, he was put into foster care. The experiences he had during his early childhood made Kevin the resilient and strong person that he is today.

Kevin graduated from the University of Kansas with a degree in Psychology. He has been practicing for 30 years before he decided to publish his first book.

Today, Kevin is well-known in his craft. He also married recently to the love of his life, Lily.